# Introduction

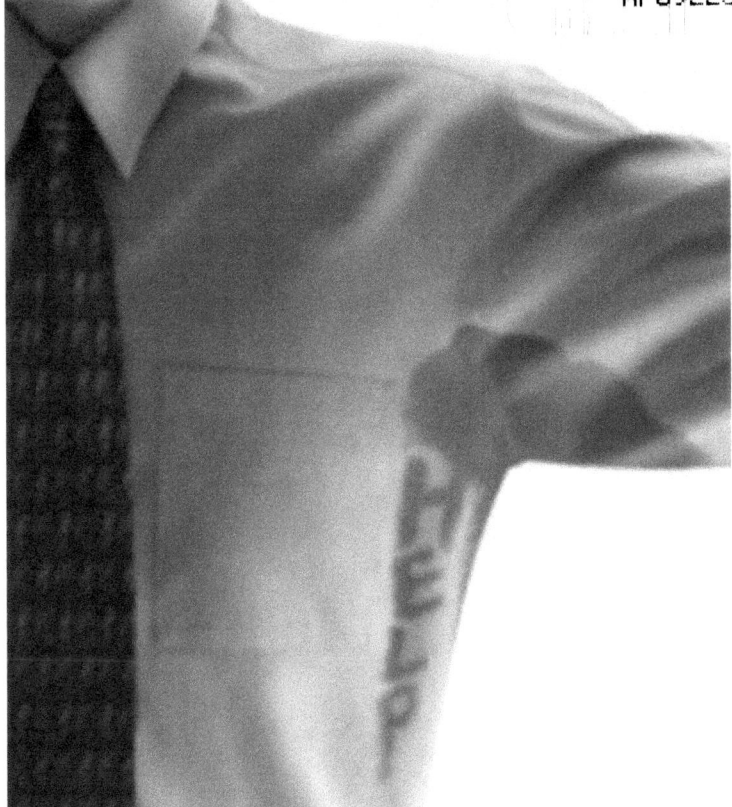

Are you sick and tired of days where you have to constantly wipe the dripping sweat from your head?

Well, I was!

Have you had enough of smelly odor problem arising from your sweating armpits?

I certainly had enough!

While every precaution has been taken in the preparation of this book, the publisher assumes no responsibility for errors or omissions, or for damages resulting from the use of the information contained herein.

SWEATING SICKNESS? HOW TO STOP SWEATING? NATURAL REMEDIES & TREATMENTS FOR EXCESSIVE SWEATING PROBLEMS

**First edition. August 1, 2017.**

Copyright © 2017 Genes Pinteles.

ISBN: 978-1386386667

Written by Genes Pinteles.

Wanna know my secret to get rid of it? These are the type of secrets you wish you knew a long time ago.

In this how to get rid of excessive sweating guide you will learn about one specific way that helped me get rid of excessive sweating for good!

Let me first introduce myself. My name is Gerard Pintellas and I was an excessive sweating sufferer, too.

Let me assure you, there are many others like you who are experiencing the same thing. In fact, a significant portion of the world population is constantly suffering from a condition called excessive sweating.

There are a few common causes of excessive sweating. The most popular one affecting most people is a medical condition is called hyperhidrosis. It is a state where you sweat more than normal and affects certain parts of your body. Most people who suffer from hyperhidrosis learn how to cure excessive sweating by visiting their doctor for professional medical advice.

From my personal experience with excessive sweating, I have been able to find out the best how to get rid of excessive sweating problems in terms of how to do it naturally, effortlessly, and painlessly and on a budget (who does not need to save some money?) and in terms of how to do it very effectively so that this type of info will help you get rid of this annoying and devastating body odor problem forever (I am talking long term solution!).

This guide shares all my secretly guarded how to get rid of this annoying body odor knowledge and know-how that I have been accumulating over the years from the pros and experts in the health and medical field.

If you just need a very quick fix (like going out for a night and impressing your partner with a very good selling body odor), I highly recommend a peek into the resources section of this book where I have listed some gold nuggets and secret resources you wish you knew before!

Just consult the resources section and these pros and experts will be able to help you and even if you are on a tight budget!

If you are on a tight budget, I am even throwing in a very valuable device for you that saves you money! (check out the Easy Skin Care Tips Device inside the book!)

The resources section contains very helpful, usable, and valuable tips and advice from the pros and it has helped me get rid of my body odor and boosted my self-confidence at the same time, too! (and again the question is who does not need a boost in self-confidence?).

The resource chapter lists the best resources that you would want to know about if you want to get rid of excessive sweating and it gives you some very valuable tips and online places to go that are going to help you. This is the type of stuff that will help you get back a nice smelling skin and body odor.

**So if you have ever experienced the following excessive sweating moments:**
 \*\* Apply antiperspirant more than once a day
 \*\* Take a shower more than once a day
 \*\* Carry undershirts to work
 \*\* Wear baggy shirts in hopes to ventilate yourself
 \*\* Wear dark colored clothes to hide your sweat stains
 \*\* Nothing you tried really works long term

**Other causes of excessive sweating also include:**
 \*\* Obesity
 \*\* The onset of puberty
 \*\* Extreme physical labor or exercises
 \*\* Extreme hot weather conditions
 \*\* Spicy or hot food
 \*\* Nervous dispositions like panic attack
 \*\* Stress
 \*\* Reaction to certain medications
 \*\* Menopause

but the good news is there are a number of ways for you to cure excessive sweating and skyrocket your self-confidence once again.

One way to cure excessive sweating is by the oral medication route where your doctor will prescribe you with medicines that promote dryness. This type of medicine will help you to sweat less however there are reports of side effects like dry mouth, palpitation and blurry vision which I can tell you from my personal experience are not fun side effects at all!

But there is one very healthy, painless, effortless and natural way that gets rid of excessive sweating for good and this is the one that I will be focusing on inside this guide because this natural way of getting rid of excessive sweating is the only one that helped me get rid of it for good!

# SWEATING SICKNESS? HOW TO STOP SWEATING? NATURAL REMEDIES & TREATMENTS FOR EXCESSIVE SWEATING PROBLEMS 3

I will tell you about my secret natural way of getting rid of excessive sweating. This type of treatment primarily involves herbs, special teas and essential oils. You are going to discover all the secret ingredients and techniques so that you can have the same results that I have achieved with this method.

**Here are sample chapters of what you are getting:**

** 9 Ways To Get Rid Of Excessive Sweating

** First Way: From Light To Heavy

** Seventh Way: The Natural Way (in my experience the only way that works long term and forever and this is basically all you need to cure your sweaty condition for good!)

** Skin Care Couponing Secrets - Easy Skin Care Tips (These are the ninja body care power tips!)

** How To Get Rid Of Excessive Sweating Resources

** Lots More

Pick up this guide to save yourself some major headache, wasted time (because I have wasted time over the years to finally get rid of this sweaty problem!), money (this one is a major problem because trying out all these non effective solutions kind of costs money, too!), stress and a

self confidence problem (because a stinky skin can get tough on you and especially if you work with clients!)

Start using your new found how to get rid of body odor forever knowledge on a regular basis and you will be able to break yourself free from spending a fortune on having to continuously invest into new excessive sweating products that might not even work!

Impress your loved ones with your good smelling and your ninja body care powers!

So, go ahead and get inside in order to get rid of your body odour forever...

## My Favorite Quote

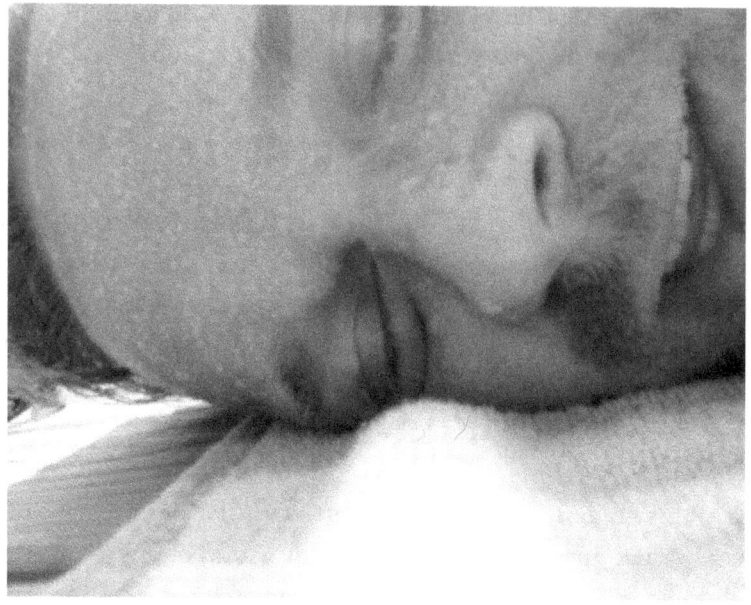

# Picture by alaspoorwho

I'm not out there sweating for three hours every day just to find out what it feels like to sweat.—Michael Jordan

# What Is Excessive Sweating

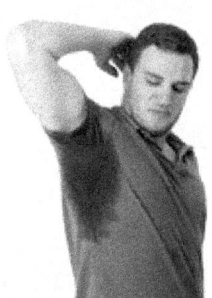

## What Exactly is Excessive Sweating and Why Are Sufferers So Desperate?

Sweat is the body's natural defense to maintain the body temperature and by sweating the body cools itself. The body cools itself of the heat which is generated due to outside temperature, physical work, and psychological stress.

Many of us suffer from over sweating ( hyperhidrosis ) or no sweating ( anhidrosis ).

Awfully enough is the fact that low sweating might be life-threatening, while over sweating may occasionally be due to some dreadful body issues.

Our body has 2 sorts of sweat glands. The eccrine sweat glands and the apocrine sweat glands. The Eccrine glands are distributed all over the body. The Apocrine sweat glands are found on the scalp, armpits and the reproductive organs. The majority of the times, it's the bacterial disintegration of sweat of both the types that produces body odor. To avoid odor due to sweat, the most practical method is to keep your skin dry.

Good cleanliness of the body won't permit bacteria to develop and multiply. Change of attire after sweating is another technique because garments carry sweat and may cause odor.

Today there are different techniques to be able to get rid of excessive sweating. These techniques include the use of antiperspirants, botox injection, Iontophoresis and in unusual cases surgery.

Sweat isn't a serious problem for the majority of us and if you are a serious excessive sweater this guide is going to help you find out about the 7 best ways how to get rid of your excessive sweating problem for good.

It's the odor that's the larger irritant, but following some simple and easy to apply techniques you will get rid of excessive sweating sooner than later.

Keep your body clean at all of the times and take basic care and you'll find the majority of the issues vanishing as you make a habit out of this. Deodorants don't reduce sweat but only mask the odor with perfume.

The requirement isn't to disguise but to stop bacterial disintegration of sweat. Exaggerated sweating, also called hyperhidrosis, may affect the whole body, but often it happens in the palms, soles, armpits, and/or groin area.

Unnecessary sweating is ordinary when someone is concerned or has a fever.

Nonetheless, when the condition is protracted, it may signal thyroid issues, low blood sugar, nerve system defects, or other medical issues.

Sweating is also called axillary hyperhidrosis in medical language and is a medical problem which is called a condition concerning dripping of sweat in the armpits, with a sustained odor.

Sweating is probably one of the most annoying kinds of hyperhidrosis, as it produces odor, which makes working in a social sector or working with clients a major problem.

The nerve system over-stimulates the sweat glands which in turn causes sweating.

The difficulty of under-arm sweating usually starts in the puberty years; nonetheless there are reported cases of kids at a younger age that are affected by this issue. The seriousness of the issue increases in youngsters, as they spend a lot of their time with their buddies at school and at playing areas.

Their pals provoke them and crack bad jokes about them which can hurt the sensation of a kid and can make an everlasting impression on their mind. This may further lead straight to withdrawal effects and social fears in the later stages of the life. Correct attention ought to be taken by moms and pops so as to make their youngsters come out of that difficulty and not have social insecurities about their future, which can hamper the character of the kid.

Sometimes elders have a tendency to reject this type of problem, and infrequently they refer to it as a cosmetic problem, when basically this is a medical problem and may be dealt with in an appropriate manner.

# What Causes Excessive Sweting?

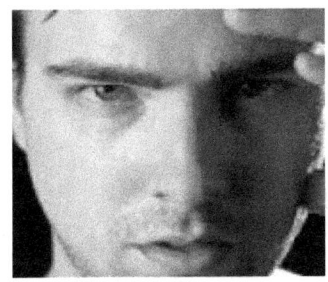

Let's look at some causes. First of all it is important to note that the cause of excessive sweating is really unknown, but in some very rare cases, Hyperhidrosis of the palms and soles is thought to be inherited like an autosomal dominant genetic trait. Many excessive sweating experts are not sure of what really causes excessive sweating and what the true roots of this nasty medical problem are.

One thing is for sure so far due to medical research Idiopathic Hyperhidrosis comes from excess sweating due to malfunction of the thyroid or pituitary gland, infection, diabetes mellitus, tumors, gout, and menopause. The disorder affects males and females in equal numbers.

In the most extreme cases, Hyperhidrosis of the palms and soles is assumed to be inherited as an autosomal dominant genetic feature.

The disorder has a bearing on females and males in equal numbers.

Excessive sweating is often caused by different factors that may cause your sweat glands to produce more sweat. Conditions such as Hyperthyrodism, fever, low blood sugar level, panic attacks etc. often cause excessive sweating in some people. These conditions often act as triggers to hyperhidrosis and therefore should be managed effectively if you hope to get rid of the condition as soon as possible.

However, the above conditions can be man managed in order to reduce their effects on the human metabolism. The following are some great treatments plus all my favorite natural remedies that have been shown very effective to get rid of excess sweating.

In my case the herbal ways have worked wonders to get rid of excessive sweating.

# Treatments - From Light To Heavy

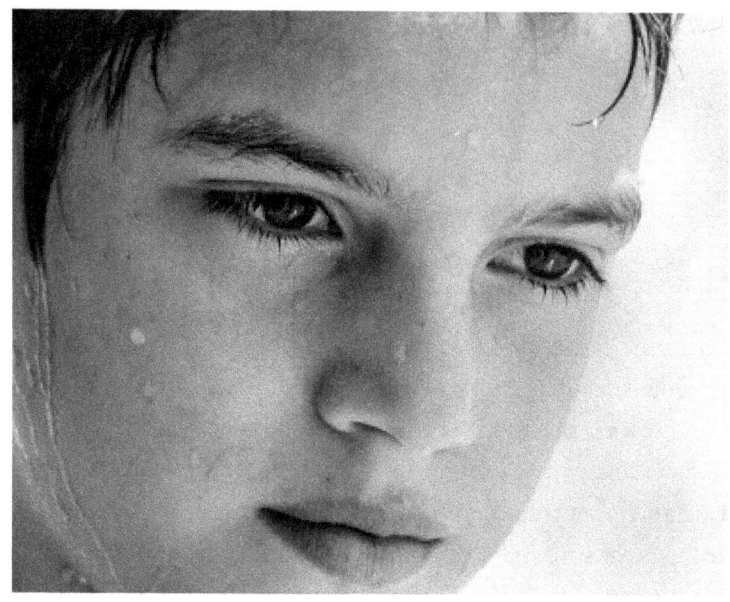

# Picture by Wilfredor

For patients with palmar-plantar-type Hyperhidrosis, cotton shoes and socks are advised.

Applications of medicated powder designed to hinder bacterial expansion is helpful.

For refractory cases, topical agents like aluminum chloride in ethyl alcohol might be indicated for axillary sweating but is usually pointless for sweating hands.

Short term courses of anticholinergic drugs are also handy in serious cases but the side-effects of dry mouth, fatigue and bowel obstruction often happen.

**Super-Antiperspirants**

Super-antiperspirants could be of some assistance. These are basically super-strength formulas of regular underarm antiperspirants. The important component, aluminum chloride basically decreases the sweat output ( unlike deodorants, which just cope with odor ).

Heavyweight formulas are available over the counter in concentrations up to twelve p.c, compared to four to six p.c in regular antiperspirants. Even stronger concentrations are available with a prescription.

Don't apply them to damaged skin or freshly shaved underarms. To extend their efficiency, apply them after sundown before bed, since the nerve system is not so active while asleep. In the morning, shower as always, then apply regular antiperspirant to the underarms.

2 or 3 applications of this mixed treatment should keep you dry for another 3 days. One approach to treatment is to govern stress. Whether psychological strain is the instigator, stress does make the sweating worse.

**Stress Control**

Doctors take 3 main approaches to help a patient calm overactive sweat glands. First is the everyday use of relaxation tapes or meditation. 2nd is biofeedback coaching; and 3rd is normal psychotherapy that investigates and hopes to take away the factors behind stress.

Surgery is available in intense cases in which sweat glands are removed from underarms, or the nerves that can trigger the sweat glands in the hands.

**Ointments or Antiperspirants**

This is the original treatment for moderate or light Hyperhidrosis. A product like Drysol is used. Doctors typically advocate applying it to areas of difficulty after drying the skin totally. Wearing it only at bedtime and then washing it off in the morning with plain water decreases the likelihood of epidermal irritation.

It is kind of annoying and will stain clothing. Don't utilize a regular deodorant later. Repeat the treatment, nightly, till the sweating is in hand. After it starts to work, use a couple of times, weekly, to maintain the effect, and utilize a regular deodorant on the other days. The medicine is less effective on the thick skin of the palms and soles.

**Oral Anticholinergic Medicine**

Certain prescription oral medicines can forestall the releasing of Acetylcholine, the neurotransmitter accountable for causing the eccrine sweat gland to go into overdrive.

Robinul is often commended and simple to take, once a day. The negative side to this drugs are the list of potential complications including dry mouth, problems with vision, trots, urinary retention and trembling.

**Astringents Conservative**

Astringent conservative treatments like Drysol and Drionics are the original treatment for Hyperhidrosis. These medicines are astringents that dry up the sweat glands.

**Topical Antiperspirants**

These agents are applied to the skin in the concerned body areas and may cause irritated skin. They're quite sloppy on clothing and sadly, have brief periods of efficiency, requiring frequent reapplications.

**Anticholinergic Medicines**

Anticholinergic medicines intend to suppress the cholinergic kick of the eccrine sweat glands by the compassionate nerve trunks to dump or reduce exaggerated sweating. Nevertheless, they could cause important unfavorable effects, limiting their value.

This is just an overview that gives you some options to choose from. The following chapters will give you some specific techniques and ways to get rid of excessive sweating for good.

Let's look at the 7 most effective ways to get rid of excessive sweating for good. I recommend to have an extra close look at the herbal way because this is how I got rid of my sweaty problem forever. The other methods are all effective as well, but some of them can have some pretty tough disadvantages and side effects and this is why I stuck to the natural way of treating my excessive sweating problem and I am using these treatment recipes religiously and the natural way works like magic.

It is in my opinion the safest, most effective and healthiest solution plus I love the long term effect of it. Some other treatments might work more in a quicker and more brutal way, but in many cases the result is just lasting for a very short term.

ter drying the skin totally. Wearing it only at bedtime and then washing it off in the morning with plain water decreases the likelihood of epidermal irritation.

It is kind of annoying and will stain clothing. Don't utilize a regular deodorant later. Repeat the treatment, nightly, till the sweating is in hand. After it starts to work, use a couple of times, weekly, to maintain the effect, and utilize a regular deodorant on the other days. The medicine is less effective on the thick skin of the palms and soles.

**Oral Anticholinergic Medicine**

Certain prescription oral medicines can forestall the releasing of Acetylcholine, the neurotransmitter accountable for causing the eccrine sweat gland to go into overdrive.

Robinul is often commended and simple to take, once a day. The negative side to this drugs are the list of potential complications including dry mouth, problems with vision, trots, urinary retention and trembling.

**Astringents Conservative**

Astringent conservative treatments like Drysol and Drionics are the original treatment for Hyperhidrosis. These medicines are astringents that dry up the sweat glands.

**Topical Antiperspirants**

These agents are applied to the skin in the concerned body areas and may cause irritated skin. They're quite sloppy on clothing and sadly, have brief periods of efficiency, requiring frequent reapplications.

**Anticholinergic Medicines**

Anticholinergic medicines intend to suppress the cholinergic kick of the eccrine sweat glands by the compassionate nerve trunks to dump or reduce exaggerated sweating. Nevertheless, they could cause important unfavorable effects, limiting their value.

This is just an overview that gives you some options to choose from. The following chapters will give you some specific techniques and ways to get rid of excessive sweating for good.

Let's look at the 7 most effective ways to get rid of excessive sweating for good. I recommend to have an extra close look at the herbal way because this is how I got rid of my sweaty problem forever. The other methods are all effective as well, but some of them can have some pretty tough disadvantages and side effects and this is why I stuck to the natural way of treating my excessive sweating problem and I am using these treatment recipes religiously and the natural way works like magic.

It is in my opinion the safest, most effective and healthiest solution plus I love the long term effect of it. Some other treatments might work more in a quicker and more brutal way, but in many cases the result is just lasting for a very short term.

# The Celebrity Way

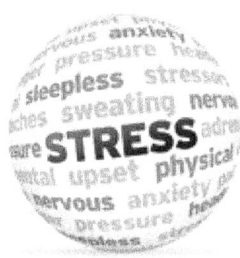

**Do you believe that BOTOX is only for the rich and famous?**

If you are really troubled with excessive sweating, Botox may be one way that you can use in order to get rid of it. You might not be famous like Paris Hilton, Angela Jolie or Jennifer Aniston, but some patients have had good successes with the Botox way.

Here are some important facts that you should consider first.

Injection of botulinum toxin (BOTOX) into the area of excessive sweating has been shown to really cause temporary relief and benefit in Hyperhidrosis.

BOTOX has the benefit that it affects nerve endings and decreases the transmission of nerve impulses to the sweat glands. This is why Botox is an effective technique in reducing the sweat production.

However on the other hand, multiple Botox injections in the palms of the hand or armpit have been described as "painful" by most patients and quite costly as most health insurance companies do not pay for these treatments. Repeated injections are nearly always required to maintain an adequate level of dryness.

In general, surgery is contemplated only when the less invasive medical treatments have failed to provide adequate treatment. This is an important point, as most insurers want documented failure of conservative therapy before endoscopic thoracic sympathectomy is approved.

Folk who find no solace from standard drug treatment for the insistent problem of sweaty palms or underarms may get short term improvement from these injections.

Botulinum poison type A is a strong chemical that in its watered down prescription form, BOTOX, has been utilized safely in treating eye muscle defects, wrinkles and other conditions.

BOTOX is nothing less than a protein that acts on the junction of the nerve and the muscle, making the muscle less active.

It decreases sweating by obstructing release of the chemical acetylcholine, which excites discharge of the sweat glands. When a touch of BOTOX is injected into the armpits or palms, it stops those areas from getting damp and sweaty.

BOTOX injections nevertheless, are only short lived and need to be repeated 2 - 3 times per year. Additionally, they're agonizing and pricey.

Some BOTOX patients say the treatment has given them replenished self confidence, while others believe the full process is not actually worth the difficulty.

Often , BOTOX injections are ineffectual in cases of serious palmar or facial Hyperhidrosis. Though alternative cures like oral medicine, BOTOX, Drysol and Drionic are available, the sole enduring, powerful treatment is to surgically stop the signal transmissions of the compassionate nerve impulse to sweat glands.

Essentially, this is achieved for all locations in the body like palms, face, armpits, and feet. This process is often known as Endoscopic Thoracoscopic Sympathectomy ( ETS ).

The most sensible person to perform Endoscopic Thoracic Sympathectomy ( ETS ) is a very highly trained, experienced, thoracic surgeon. The operation is performed on an outpatient basis while patient is under general anesthesia administered by a board-certified or board-eligible anesthesiologist.

The considerate nerves are found along the back, just behind the ribs. The surgeon uses a scope with magnification and illumination supplied by the camera to view the considerate nerves. The vascular surgeon cuts or clamps the compassionate nerves of the ganglion through 2 little cuts ( five to ten mm ) below the armpit area on every side of the chest.

In the cutting system, the nerve is just cut. These nerves are cut to stop or cut back the body's capability to produce sweat in those identified areas of difficulty. Our surgeons opt for this methodology over the clamping technique. The clipping technique can most likely result in lower success rates if the clip migrates from the nerve on is applied too loosely. The process is performed bilaterally in the same session. After patients wake up from the anesthesia, they're moved to a recovery room, where they're punctiliously monitored, before getting discharged to go back home.

Patients can return to work or college inside a couple of days. The process is intensely effective for palmar and axillary Hyperhidrosis. The endoscopic method is really safe and is curative in 98% of patients. The number one indication for surgery was palmar Hyperhidrosis ( PH ) in 302 of 309 patients ( 97.7% ), though in seven patients ( 2.3% ) axillary Hyperhidrosis ( AH ) was the main indication.

A family history was brought about in 74 of 132 ( 56.01% ) and a provocative reply to hand lotion was present in 101 of 132 ( 76.5% ). Thoracoscopic sympathectomy afforded just about immediate cures for PH, with major enhancement in a hundred percent for whom the sympathectomy was done. Of 180 patients prospectively queried in detail, 173 ( 96.1% ) had some quantity of plantar Hyperhidrosis. Of these, 148 ( 84.4% ) had some improvement, with seventy ( 40.5% ) achieving complete relief of the plantar Hyperhidrosis. In 98 patients who had some grumbles of AH, 68 ( 69.4% ) were utterly relieved with the AH, while twenty-five ( 25.5% ) were relieved though not utterly cured.

In seven patients, the main indication for sympathectomy was AH and of these, three ( 42.9% ) had complete relief, two ( 28.6% ) had partial relief, and two ( 28.6% ) had no relief. Of the whole series of 309 patients, four ( 1.3% ) developed grim compensatory Hyperhidrosis ( CH ). In 180 prospectively queried patients, CH was present in 81 ( forty five percent ).

# The Surgical Way

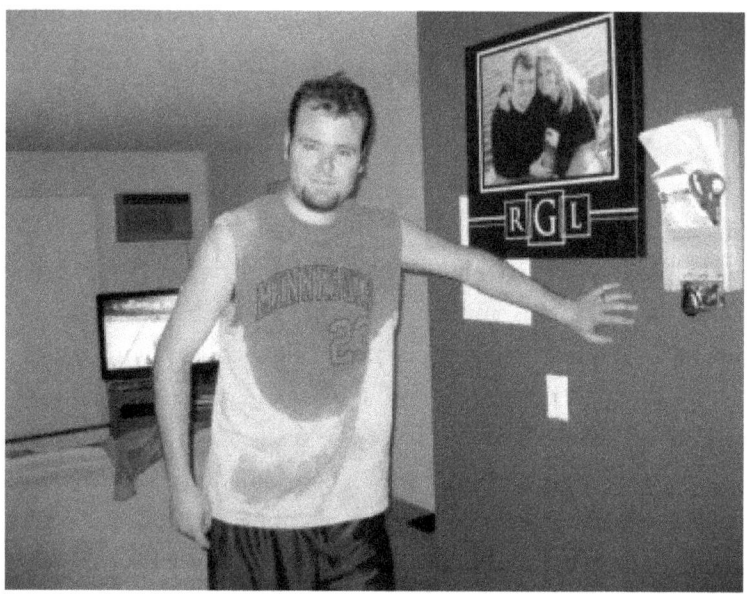

Hyperhidrosis surgery has come a ways in the decade. Historically , enormous cuts were made in the chest to surgically interrupt the considerate trunk, all to attempt to treat Hyperhidrosis.

With the appearance of minimally aggressive systems to work in the chest through endoscopes and surgical instruments, a process has appeared that's very impressive in treating patients with sweating of the hands, underarms, face, scalp as well as patients that have facial blushing. This is the most sturdy treatment for Hyperhidrosis.

Clipping the thoracic considerate trunk at the correct levels will instantly eliminate Hyperhidrosis. It is sort of dramatic to see a patient wake up from anesthesia and to pay attention to a dry hand or axilla. With alteration of the level of sympathectomy, compensatory Hyperhidrosis is also minimized or eliminated.

## The Iontopheresis Way

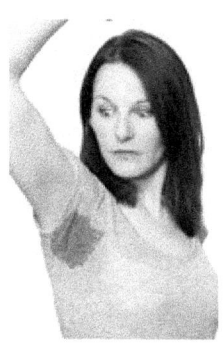

This treatment consists of the following. The iontopheresis way consists of electrical stimulation of the affected areas. The site of the patient's choice is submerged in water and electricity is emitted by the iontopheresis device.

The intensity is then gradually increased until the patient notices a tingling feeling, which some patients find unpleasant. After several uses, the patient will sweat less for four to six weeks.

To really get it to work, the iontopheresis way needs to be used one half hour every night, per site.

This iontopheresis treatment is repeated until the sweating is well under control.

Drionic® is the product recommended. The results may vary: in cases of light Hyperhidrosis, some patients are happy, but others may consider the treatment too time-consuming and expensive.

# The Herbal Way 1

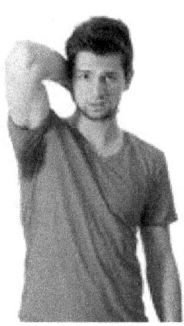

The herbal way is the way how I treated my excessive sweating problem for good. I will be showing you 5 specific herbal ways that you can apply ASAP and if you apply them religiously like I do, you will have very good results.

The advantages of herbal treatments are huge because they are the safest, healthiest, most effective and the least expensive. In addition they are painless and long lasting. Other treatments are very painful and have to be repeated in order to be long term effective.

If you are suffering from unrestrained sweating way beyond what the body must do to govern body temperature, my favorite technique that I call the herbal way of getting rid of sweating might be of interest to you.

Don't we hate this moisture laying on the surface of our skin rather than evaporating like it typically would.

I hear that some sufferers even have issues with grip due to near-permananet wet hands and others have to have one or two changes of clothing everyday.

As I told you before, none of these non herbal other treatments that I discussed above are without hazards and all are really costly. Their efficiency also appears to alter from one patient to another and horrific stories are common.

Especially associated with the surgical option ( which needs each lung to be slumped in turn to reach the nerves in the chest hole)

This is why the herbal way is my favorite way of getting rid of sweat forever!

# SWEATING SICKNESS? HOW TO STOP SWEATING? NATURAL REMEDIES & TREATMENTS FOR EXCESSIVE SWEATING PROBLEMS

The herbal way is the way that has helped me get rid of my excessive sweating for good and it has changed my life forever.

Let's get started with the herbal way of treating excessive sweating.

This is a completely natural, risk free treatment concerning a cheap kitchen herb.

I hope that you will appreciate this easy yet effective technique.

The herb in query has basically been medically proven, too.

The treatment was evaluated by a medical grouping of analysts at the College of Medication, Isfahan School of Medical Sciences in Iran and it is an easy "tea" solution made of the dried leaves of a standard herb, and water.

In the medical study, thirty-five patients ( eighteen men and seventeen girls, aged 8-49 years ) who'd been diagnosed as having either palmar or plantar ( hand or foot ) hyperhidrosis were given the treatments 3 times per day for 6 weeks.

The solution was simply applied to the skin ( they did not drink it ) where unjustifiable sweating was an issue.

After 6 weeks of this treatment the people in the study who received the tea experienced seriously more alleviation from their sweating than the people that were given a fake pill.

In reality the solution was shown to reduce sweating in the hands, feet and under arms by as much as 37% on account of the herb's acid properties. These are the directions if you would like to make the solution at home.

Use 3 spoons of dried leaves combined with two hundred and fifty ml ( 8.5 oz ) of room temperature water and leave to steep for twenty-four to forty eight hours.

After straining, the ensuing solution can be applied to underarms, feet or hands.

The analysts also suggest another treatment for plantar hyperhidrosis which influences the bottoms of the feet.

They like to recommend a dry powder of the herb, placed in the shoes. The powder can be manufactured by grinding dried leaves with an electronic or hand mill. The solution or powder should be applied to the trouble spot 3 times per day and the area should be fully dried before application.

# The Herbal Way 2

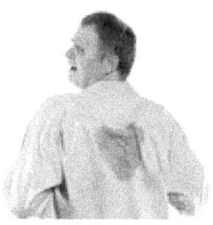

**Sage Tea Remedy**

Sage Tea is an excellent remedy for the pesky and embarrassing situation of hyper-sweating.

Since sage is not particularly appealing to the palette it is flavored with chamomile tea to make the concoction more palatable. This herbal sage and chamomile extract has to be prepared each morning and the herbal formulation can start showing results in three weeks time. Chamomile is a tasty herbal tea and thus makes it quite appealing to a lot of people. The recipe to share for the same is as follows.

**Ingredients**

1 teaspoon fresh or dried sage leafes
1 1/2 tablespoons of Chamomile petals
1 cup of water

**Instructions:**

Bring the water to a boiling temperature and remove it from the heat.

Add both ingredients chamomile and sage to the water and cover it with a lid.

Let the whole concoction stand and steep for approximately 15 minutes.

Pass the resultant liquid through a mesh strainer straight into your favorite cup. You may enjoy the preparation as it is or you can add a bit of honey and lemon to enhance the taste to your liking.

**Alternative Way:**

Another way which is fast and easy. Take approximately 8 oz of water and add 2 or 3 drops of sage extract to it, additionally you may add one or two teaspoon's of apple-cider vinegar, which is known to help reduce high amount of sweating. Though this method is high on convenience, you need to exercise caution with this approach.

At any given point in time you can only take this sage extract for 3 to 4 weeks at a stretch, then you have to let it go for sometimes before resuming the consumption of this preparation.

In females it has been shown to result in heavy vaginal bleeding if too much of it taken for a long period of time. It also puts you on the risk of excessive high bleeding in case you get injured.

The best way to go about combating the menace of excessive perspiration is to go for a combination of herbal remedies.

You may go for an internal remedy and pair it with the use of a really effective natural antiperspirant.

Again you have a choice between an over the counter formulation which certainly has ingredients which may cause undesired side-effects like Alzheimer's disease, cancer, or various blood diseases.

You suffer from a chronic condition and it is best to avoid excessive exposure to these undesired chemicals as far as possible which can pose a health hazard and be risky for you in the long run.

Here, I will show you how to make a natural antiperspirant at a fraction of the cost of a commercial formulation without the attendant side effects.

Here is a tried and tested recipe for you, take a bowl and mix the powders i.e.

- 2 tablespoons of alum
- 1/4 cup baking soda
- 1/4 cup corn starch
- add 2 to 3 drops of tea tree oil
- some coconut oil
- and 4-5 drops of any essential oil of your choice.

Mix well and transfer into an empty antiperspirant container.
Oils of choice could be lavender, vanilla, sandalwood, or maybe rose.

# The Herbal Way 3

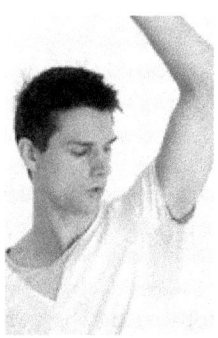

Have you ever imagined stretching your hand to shake the hand of a person who has sweaty palms. Indeed it can be really embarrassing and quite a turn off.

The following are some great natural remedies that have been shown to get rid of excess sweating. Indeed they work wonders for most people who have hyperhidrosis.

**Tea Tree Oil**

Tea tree oil has been used for ages as a way of getting rid of hyperhidrosis. It is quite a powerful anti bacterial which will not only kill germs but also makes you feeling very refreshed.

The tea tree oil has quite a number of uses from its health benefits to skin care benefits.

This is a must use for any person dealing with this condition.

Tea tree oil has been used for ages as a way of getting rid of hyperhidrosis. It is quite a powerful anti bacterial which will not only kill germs but has a revitalizing aspect to it.

The tea tree oil has quite a number of uses from its health benefits to skin care benefits. This is a must use for any person dealing with the condition of excessive sweating.

**Burdock**

I strongly recommend the use of Burdock which is a know blood purifier and helps the body in ridding it of fluids and toxins through urination. Get a bottle from a health food store and follow the directions.

Burdock is also a very powerful herb that works wonders. The herb helps the body get rid of excess sweat through other different avenues thus helping you sweat less. Such avenues include the lymph, kidney or colon. It offers very good results however it is quite bitter hence requires a lot of courage on the part of its user.

A word of caution here, excessive use can have a mild laxative effect, too!

**Sage**

It is known as an antiperspirant that is widely found in most parts of the world. You can choose to grind it and take it with tea or chose to apply it as a cream on your skin.

Sage does help reduce excess weight and has had a quite a large number of positive review from happy users.

As you can see you do not have to suffer from hyperhidrosis as the above natural remedies have helped very many people get rid of this embarrassing condition.

It is however important to seek the help of a professional professional dermatologist before you choose to use any of these natural products as your skin might react negatively to them.

Since underlying conditions such as stress and low blood sugar can make the condition worse, it is also important that you take control of these underlying triggers, too.

With the right choices you are sure to get rid of this condition and live a happier, healthy and sweat-free life.

## The Herbal Arjuvedic Way 4

**Ingredients and Instructions:**

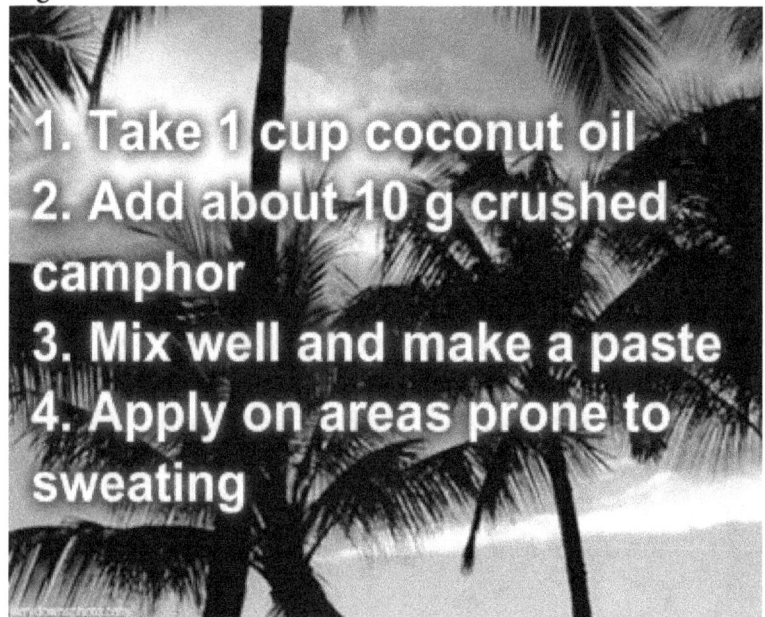

1. Take 1 cup coconut oil
2. Add about 10 g crushed camphor
3. Mix well and make a paste
4. Apply on areas prone to sweating

**More How To Stop Excessive Sweating Tips - The Ajurvedic Way:**

These remedies are based on the principles of the Ajurvedic science. Ajurveda is the ancient Indian science of healing. Ajurveda is a completely non-invasive, and natural way and the Ajurvedic recipes can be prepared at home.

Below you will find some basic Ajurvedic techniques for excessive sweating that will be very effective if repeated on a daily basis.

Please, consult your doctor if your symptoms persist.

# SWEATING SICKNESS? HOW TO STOP SWEATING? NATURAL REMEDIES & TREATMENTS FOR EXCESSIVE SWEATING PROBLEMS

Drink 1 Cup Of Tomatoe Juice Every Day
- rich in Anti-Oxidants
- helps regulate sweat glands
Keep Body cool!
- eat fresh grapes
- drink up to 10 glasses fresh spring water every day

# 25 Quick Tips How To Stop Sweating

1. Drink a lot of water - hydration keeps body temperatures low and therefore less sweat will be produced. Water is vital to life. It effectively flushes out excess minerals and pushes out all toxins and waste products. The experts recommend six to eight glasses of water everyday.

2. Stay Calm - stress and nervousness instantly triggers the sweat glands.

3. Cut down your caffeine intake - caffeine tends to cause anxiety which in return triggers the body to excessive sweating.

4. Acupuncture - this simple ancient technique works like gangbusters. It simply targets certain body parts to balance energy and also relax the brain by controlling the hypothalamus which goes down to reduce sweat.

5. Yoga - one of the best natural ways to control excessive sweating. This works through meditation, calming down the nerves and subsequently lessening sweat production. Since Yoga teaches proper breathing, it works well especially when one is stressed or uneasy.

6. Avoid using deodorant or soap - this may come as a surprise but unknown to most people, the effects of deodorants or soaps not compatible with your body will do you more harm than good. They cause more bacteria to build up on the skin, which end up setting foul odor. That's why it's important to choose a deodorant or soap that suits your body.

# SWEATING SICKNESS? HOW TO STOP SWEATING? NATURAL REMEDIES & TREATMENTS FOR EXCESSIVE SWEATING PROBLEMS

7. Take a cold shower - Ok, you won't like this. In spite of the uncomfortable effects of a cold shower, it surely works wonders. While you are at it, try using an antibacterial soap to ensure the body is clean and odor-free.

8. Avoid taking hot baths - while baths may be useful in eliminating toxins through increased body temperature, problems of excessive sweating outweigh their benefits.

9. Drink tomato juice - To be honest, I love this and I know it helps. The extra vitamins and nutrients come in mighty handy.

10. Avoid Hot drinks - when it comes to excessive sweating, these are your worst enemies, and that includes hot coffee too. Imagine the effect they give if you are just about to go for an important meeting or make a presentation. So why not try going for juice, lemonade or iced-beverages to regulate your temperature.

11. Drink sage tea - Taking these herbs two to four times a day keeps the body functioning well as well regulating sweat production.

12. Boil tea bags then soak your hands and feet in them! - A useful but rather questionable home made remedy to control excessive armpit sweating.

13. Rub the armpits with wool pads soaked in a mixture of baking soda and lemon juice

14. Avoid alcohol, cigarettes and drugs - An absolute no-brainer. These chemicals make it harder for the body to control sweating because they cause a delay in blood circulation.

15. Avoid spicy, sugary and chemically-processed foods.

Spicy foods may be tasty, delightful and healthy, but they make your body sweat on a more frequently basis and in very short time periods. Large intakes of chemical toxins will aggravate sweating, too.

Same for high fructose syrup used by some brands to sweeten food. Do not use any pre-made, packaged, frozen, greasy, ready-to-eat and fast foods because these foods make the problem worse.

16. Eat the "healthy" foods. Food with fewer complex B vitamins means that your body cannot allow for an efficient absorption of nutrients and a proper break down of the toxins and body waste.

This in turn means a strained body which leads to more sweaty moments. What foods should you take then?
a. Whole grains - sources of B Vitamins and fiber.
b. Fresh Fruits - whatever you like, they should form a crucial component in your daily eating habits. Any will do from apples, oranges, raisins, melon, peaches, watermelons, blueberries, strawberries, plums, etc. You could try taking a fruits for breakfast or as a healthy snack.
c. Vegetables - Salads and vegetables are an excellent source of B Vitamins.
d. Proteins - Fish, eggs and a little bit of red meat. As for vegetarians, beans will do a great job. Avoid andy type of deep-fried foods.

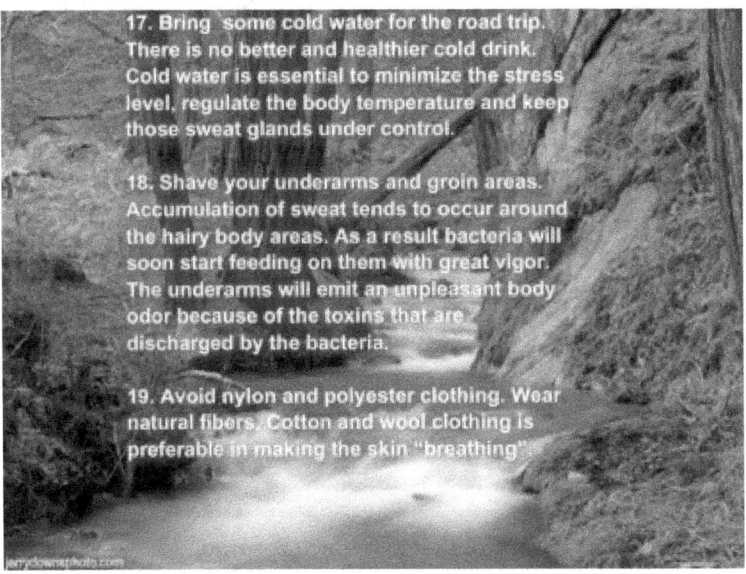

17. Bring some cold water for the road trip. There is no better and healthier cold drink. Cold water is essential to minimize the stress level, regulate the body temperature and keep those sweat glands under control.

18. Shave your underarms and groin areas. Accumulation of sweat tends to occur around the hairy body areas. As a result bacteria will soon start feeding on them with great vigor. The underarms will emit an unpleasant body odor because of the toxins that are discharged by the bacteria.

19. Avoid nylon and polyester clothing. Wear natural fibers. Cotton and wool clothing is preferable in making the skin "breathing".

20. Wear loose fitting shirts. If your clothes are too tight, you are depriving your body enough air to circulate around it. This condition increases sweating. It triggers the sweat glands to produce more sweat. Keep your collar open during extreme hot weather conditions. Simply wear light clothing like a Tshirt and skirt/pants.

Carry an extra shirt all the time. Be smart and keep a change of clothing items during hot days.

22. Wear underwear. High quality undershirts that are made out of cotton or just a plain Tshirt to absorb the body sweat.

23. Starching your clothing prevents it from sticking to your body. This will help keep the body cool.

24. Keeping your head cool when you are exposed to the sun for long time. A hat and glasses are a good idea. Shades help protect your eyes from the bright light and heat. Go for sunglasses with reflective coating and polarized lenses.

25. Wearing socks helps keep the feet cooler. They absorb feet perspiration and help with faster evaporation.

## Next Steps

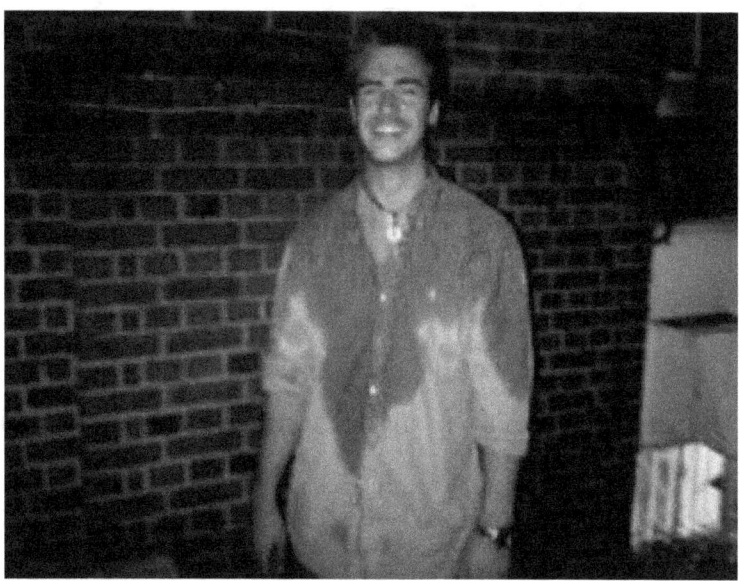

Just go to this appropriate section of the book to find the specific information. You will become better and better at this and soon you will be a true skin expert yourself.

Once you feel ready and have absorbed enough information, it is time to get into the practical phase. You can always come back to the researching and learning phase in order to develop more skills and expertise as you go.

Now, it is time for you to go ahead and pick your favorite way of getting rid of excessive sweating. Once you decided what way to pick, you can go ahead and get started with the physical phase of the process.

If you still need some more information in order to get started with the specific way that you picked, I highly recommend to you to dig deeper into the research about that specific way and seek more professional advice and tips that you can add to the process.

As you go through the research phase, you will be able to identify an expert who can point you into the right direction depending on your chosen way and your personal situation, lifestyle and goal.

Once you are done with the research, you can go ahead and pick one way as a starting point.

I started with the natural way myself and this is how I got rid of excessive sweating forever so I highly recommend to go with the natural way first.

You can always do more research later. The important thing is to pick one way or several ways (but never pick more than 2 ways at the same time because too much might overwhelm you) and get started with the process as soon as possible.

I hope that you are informed, encouraged and motivated enough in order to get started, and I hope you will achieve a sweat-free lifestyle like I have been able to achieve it with the natural way.

I was able to achieve it by using the natural ingredients and recipes that I included in the natural way part of this book.

It is up to you to identify and pick your own favorite way. Go ahead and use the way or ways that you like to use as a starting point and go from there. You can always adjust and make changes as you go.

Do it right now and change your sweaty lifestyle into a healthy, happy, sweat-free and socially enjoyable lifestyle that you enjoy today.

To your success without sweaty skin!

**Additional Resources**

http://www.howcast.com/videos/397906-Quick-Tips-How-to-Stop-Sweating-So-Much

http://www.ehow.com/how_5306215_stop-sweating-much.html

http://www.dailymotion.com/video/xt8fxn_how-to-stop-sweating-so-much-on-face_shortfilms

http://forumhealthcare.org/how-to-stop-sweating-so-much-t45173.html[1]

http://health.howstuffworks.com/skin-care/underarm-care/problems/excessive-underarm-sweating3.htm

http://www.herbnet.com/ask%20the%20herbalist/asktheherbalist_excessive_sweating.htm[2]

http://www.youtube.com/watch?v=Vr48Z6U9-9c

---

1. http://www.dailymotion.com/video/xt8fxn_how-to-stop-sweating-so-much-on-face_shortfilms
2. http://health.howstuffworks.com/skin-care/underarm-care/problems/excessive-underarm-sweating3.htm

# Skin Care Quiz

**Excessive Sweating Quiz**

| C | X | I | R | W | O | D | O | R | L | B | W | V | S | W |
|---|---|---|---|---|---|---|---|---|---|---|---|---|---|---|
| A | C | C | L | I | M | A | T | I | S | A | T | I | O | N |
| M | V | R | Q | R | P | H | E | R | O | M | O | N | E | S |
| Q | T | R | A | N | S | P | I | R | A | T | I | O | N | Y |
| P | E | R | S | P | I | R | A | T | I | O | N | D | E | N |
| A | Q | J | A | N | H | I | D | R | O | S | I | S | S | Q |
| D | N | B | C | W | S | W | E | A | T | I | N | G | B | S |
| H | Y | P | E | R | H | I | D | R | O | S | I | S | M | C |
| I | H | Q | T | E | M | P | E | R | A | T | U | R | E | I |
| H | N | C | M | N | E | O | L | V | G | K | P | E | A | O |

**Excessive Sweating Quiz**

# Quiz Answers

1. Transpiration
2. Hyperhidrosis
3. Odor
4. Temperature
5. Anhidrosis
6. Sweating
7. Perspiration
8. Pheromones
9. Acclimatisation

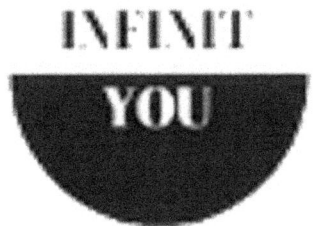

## About the Publisher

InfinitYou is a hybrid general interest trade publisher. One of the first of its kind InfinitYou publishes physical books, electronic books, and audiobooks in various genres. Our publications are meant to educate, edify and entertain readers of all walks of life from babies to the elderly.

Home to more than twenty imprints such as Infinit Baby, Infinit Kids, Infinit Girl, Infinit Boy, Infinit Coloring, Infinit Swear Words, Infinit Activities, Infinit Productivity, Infinit Cat, Infinit Dog, Infinit Love, Infinit Family, Infinit Survival, Infinit Health, Infinit Beauty, Infinit Spirituality, Infinit Lifestyle, Infinit Wealth, Infinit Romance, and lots more.

www.ingramcontent.com/pod-product-compliance
Lightning Source LLC
LaVergne TN
LVHW020456080526
838202LV00057B/5981